Psychiatric Assessment

Forensic Focus
Edited by Murray Cox

This series takes the currently crystallizing field of Forensic Psychotherapy as its focal point, offering a forum for the presentation of theoretical and clinical issues. It will also embrace such influential neighbouring disciplines as language, law, literature, criminology, ethics and philosophy, as well as psychiatry and psychology, its established progenitors.

Forensic Focus series

Forensic Psychotherapy
Crime, Psychodynamics and the
Offender Patient
Edited by Christopher Cordess
and Murray Cox
Forewords by John Gunn
and Richard Wells
ISBN 1 85302 240 4
Forensic Focus 1

The Cradle of Violence
Essays on Psychiatry, Psychoanalysis and
Literature
Stephen Wilson
ISBN 1 85302 306 X
Forensic Focus 2

A Practical Guide to Forensic
 Psychotherapy
Edited by Estela V. Welldon
and Cleo Van Velsen
Forewords by Fiona Caldicott, DBE
and Helena Kennedy QC
ISBN 1 85302 389 2
Forensic Focus 3

Challenges in Forensic
Psychotherapy
Edited by Hjalmar van Marle
and Wilma van den Berg
ISBN 1 85302 419 8
Forensic Focus 5

Remorse and Reparation
Edited by Murray Cox
ISBN 1 85302 452 X
ISBN 1 85302 451 1
Forensic Focus 7

of related interest

The Assessment of Criminal
Behaviour of Clients in Secure
Settings
Edited by Mary McMurran and John Hodge
ISBN 1 85302 124 5

Forensic Focus 8

Psychiatric Assessment

Pre and Post Admission Assessment

A series of assessments designed for professionals working
with mentally disordered offenders and clients
with challenging behaviours

Valerie A. Brown

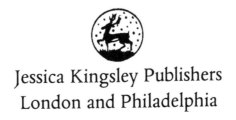

Jessica Kingsley Publishers
London and Philadelphia

First published in the United Kingdom in 1998 by
Jessica Kingsley Publishers Ltd
116 Pentonville Road
London N1 9JB, England
and
1900 Frost Road, Suite 101
Bristol, PA 19007, U S A

Copyright © 1998 Valerie A. Brown

Library of Congress Cataloging in Publication Data
A CIP catalogue record for this book is available from the Library of Congress

British Library Cataloguing in Publication Data
Brown, Valerie Anne
Psychiatric assessment: pre and post admission.
(Forensic Focus; 8)
1. Mental illness – Diagnosis I. Title
616.8'9'075
ISBN 1 85302 575 5

ISBN 1-85302-575-5

Printed and Bound in Great Britain by
Athenaeum Press, Gateshead, Tyne & Wear

Contents

Parts 1 to 10 must be completed during the pre-admission assessment. Highlighted parts must be addressed during the pre-admission assessment if applicable to the individual.

Acknowledgements

I would like to thank all of those colleagues who gave their time and expertise over the last four years, in particular those who helped put this series of assessments into use and came back with positive comments and constructive criticism, including Lucy Hamilton, Sue Iles, Tony Lingiah, Anne Pirie, Rob Pollock and Iris Wright.

I want to thank David and Julie Stanford for the production of all the drafts, and my husband Steve for his patience and support.

In memory of Dr Murray Cox, without whose enthusiasm and support I might never have had the courage to submit the manuscript.

Introduction

This series of assessments has been designed to provide a clear focus on key elements in the assessment of mentally disordered offenders and those with extremely challenging behaviours. The guiding philosophy is to provide the practitioner with a tool that will capture essential and relevant information to enable care teams to develop a comprehensive management strategy.

A core skill required by the practitioner is that of objectivity. These assessments are objective. This ensures that the information collated relates to evidence found in the individual's background. The evidence demonstrates the severity and frequency of particular elements and any of the changes found in their life and subsequent behaviour.

I work as a team leader on the women's admission assessment unit in Broadmoor Hospital. Four years ago I began to look at a variety of assessment tools. After reviewing a great number of options it was apparent that forensic assessments needed to reflect forensic issues. This series of assessments is the culmination of a working process that developed tools to assess specific aspects and behaviours.

These tools are not definitive – every new assessment can identify other areas of concern not currently covered; however, the format allows and encourages additions to the tools.

Instructions for use

- Read and make sure you understand each section before use.
- Use the title of each assessment as a heading and keep the information specific to the part.
- It is recommended that all shaded areas within each assessment are completed: this provides base-line information.
- The assessments highlighted are those covering risk issues and are only required to be completed if there is a history of the subject. It is important to understand that although you may not have any information relating to these areas, this must not be taken as evidence that the subjects are not relevant
- Note names of anyone who may be referred to for further detail.
- Always check frequency and severity of identified issues: these are vital for risk assessment.
- Watch for non-verbal communication; identify any changes in behaviour with the subject under discussion.
- Take advice on whether to interview alone.
- Bear in mind that informal interviews are often more productive than question and answer sessions.
- Advise the current care team of any information you have given to the individual.
- In the formal report it is appropriate to recommend further assessment if required. This could relate to a specific issue, for example learning disabilities.
- The only place for opinion is at the conclusion of the report. The main body of the report should reflect what is found or, equally important, what is not found at the time of the assessment. There may not be evidence to reflect an issue; the report should state this rather than assume the issue does not exist.

SUGGESTED REPORT FORMAT

Name:.....................................   Date of birth: ....

Current legal status: ....   Current location: ....

Name of assessor:..........................   Name of person referring: ....

Assessed on:.................................   Time of assessment: ....

Reason for referral:...

....

The report should give each assessment heading followed by the information found. In the event of there being nothing found, the report should state this.

At the bottom of the report all sources of information should be identified and finally recommendations or opinions stated. These could include a recommendation for a specialised assessment by another assessor

The following sample is of a 12 month to view chart which can be used to report rapidly the frequency of a particular behaviour; for example, deliberate self harm with the corresponding letter to signify category and number to signify severity, eg. A4 (see Part 15).

Assessment for:...........................

Name:...............................   Date of birth: Sex: M/F

YEAR	Jan	Feb	Mar	Apr	May	Jun	Jul	Aug	Sep	Oct	Nov	Dec
1												
2												
3												
4												

Part 1: Basic Care Issues

First language	spoken/signed
Requires interpreter	
What (if any) language is the individual most literate in?	(specify)
Current MHA section	
Orientated in	person, place, time

Staff report

- probable hallucinations
- delusions
- obsessive/compulsive behaviour
- panic attacks
- depressive episodes
- elated episodes

Individual reports

- hallucinations
- obsessive/compulsive behaviour
- depressive episodes
- elated episodes
- anxiety

1

The individual is known to have epilepsy with	petit mal /grand mal seizures
Seizures are believed to be hysterical	yes/no
Does the individual use coping mechanisms?	(specify)
It is known that the individual has used controlled/ 'recreational' drugs	yes/no
It is believed that the individual has used controlled/ 'recreational' drugs	yes/no
The individual has admitted having used controlled/ 'recreational' drugs	yes/no
How were drugs used?	own/shared needles
It is believed that the individual has abused	alcohol/aerosols/solvents
It is known that the individual has abused	alcohol/aerosols/solvents
Does the individual smoke?	average number in 24 hours

Is the patient compliant with treatment?	always/usually/rarely
Has a second opinion been	• requested • granted/refused (specify) • date of certificate
Suffers from motion sickness	yes/no
Does the individual require prompting assistance with their personal hygiene?	(specify)
Are there any difficulties/ problems relating to	bladder/bowels/mobility
Has the individual seen a continence adviser/other nurse specialist?	
Do they have	dentures/hearing aid(s)/contact lenses/glasses/any other prosthesis (specify)
Does the individual practise their	religious beliefs/cultural beliefs/ personal beliefs
Does the individual require any specific considerations in order to practise any belief?	

Can these needs be met by contracts/facilities within the hospital?	e.g.: diet/religious adviser/ privacy at set times
Do they have specific	cultural needs/dietary needs that require arranging prior to admission
What is the individual's view regarding	• referral to special hospital • index offence (if applicable) • self harm (if applicable) • violence towards others/self

Part 2: Medical History

Physical illness(es)

Known allergy(ies)

Has the individual had any of these tests in the past 12 months?

FBC   ESR   U & E   TFT   LFT

Hepatitus B   HIV   Hormones   Sickle cell

any other blood test(s)

Clozaril/lithium levels

Anti-convulsant levels
Other prescribed drug levels
Tests for non-prescribed drugs

Chest X-ray
Other X-ray(s)

Electro encephalogram
Electro cardiogram

MRI scan
CT scan

Mammogram/cervical smear/ hysterectomy

Testicular/prostrate gland health checks

Sterilisation	how/when/where
Out patient appointment	• nature of appointment • treatment • reason for treatment • with whom • where • when
Contraception	• IUD • Depot injection • oral • hormone therapy/contraceptive pill
Implants	• hormone • pace-maker • other (specify)
Transplanted organ	(specify)
If the individual has a medical condition, e.g. diabetes, do they	• believe this • accept this • have insight into the condition • and its potential

Part 3: Incident History

Breaking windows
- with hand(s)
- by other means (specify)

Throwing
- objects
- cutlery
- hot/corrosive fluids
- furniture inc: TV/VCR/music centres

Upturning furniture including TV/VCR/music centre

yes/no

Assaulted
- family
- patient/inmate
- nursing staff
- medical staff
- custody staff
- other staff (specify)
- stranger
  - male
  - female
  - adult(s) (specify age)
  - child(ren) (specify age)

Injury caused to	

- family
- patient/inmate
- nursing staff
- medical staff
- custody staff
- other staff (specify)
  - male
  - female
  - adult(s) (specify age)
  - child(ren) (specify age)

Assaulted victim(s)	

- from the front
- from behind
- with a weapon (specify)
- by strangulation
- by biting
- by kicking
- by punching
- by slapping
- by scratching
- by spitting
- by pulling hair
- by any other means (specify)

Assault(s) specifically targeted	

neck/face/eyes

Assault(s) took place in	• the individual's home
	• previous placement
	• current placement
	• residential setting
	• custodial setting
	• public place, e.g. street/park/building
	• hospital
	• special hospital

Does the individual give reason(s) for the assault(s)?	(specify)

Incident(s) behaviour	• acts alone
	• acts with others
	• encourages others

Part 4: External network

Number of children

Name(s) of child(ren)

Location of child(ren)

foster parents/local authority care/other relative/adopted (specify)

Social worker(s)

Child(ren) are on 'at risk' register

Specific court instructions *re* access

Telephone/visits/letters to child(ren), give details including

who dials/how often/what time/day/who checks/who arranges visits/transport/ funding/frequency of letters

Age(s) of child(ren) when separated

Length of separation

Statutory benefits

who holds pension/benefit books

Pensions

Court of Protection

is the individual's financial management under the CoP

External agency(ies)/contact(s)

- psychiatric consultant(s)
- probation/parole officer(s)
- Home Office contract(s)
- social worker(s)
- rehabilitation officer(s)
- social services
- other (specify)

Housing issues

- county council
- housing authority
- privately owned
- rented
- other (specify)

Is the individual receiving housing benefits?

Direct family members/ significant others

- in prison
- in hospital
- in care
- known to social services
- known to the police

Does current care team maintain contact/access with hospital/prison etc?

yes/no

Part 5: Behaviour at Night

Night sedation prescribed	detail(s)
Night sedation regularly used	detail(s)
Night sedation refused	
Night sedation used occasionally	
Aggressive following sedation	form of aggression (specify)
Smokes in lounge	yes/no
Watches television	own/communal
Talks to	staff/other residents
Reads in	own room/lounge
Writes in	own room/lounge
Listens to	radio/cassettes/records/CDs
Goes to room/to sleep	usual time(s)
Does the individual sleep	usually well/fitfully
Does the individual complain about their sleeping pattern?	(specify)

Does the individual sleep with

- light(s) on/light(s) off
- television/radio on

Changes into night attire	yes/no
Sleeps fully dressed	yes/no

Sleeps

- under bedclothes
- on top of bedclothes
- makes up bed on the floor

Wakes for

- drink
- cigarette

Incontinent of

urine often/rarely
faeces often/rarely

Appears to have/complains of having

- nightmares
- vivid dreams
- 'flashbacks' asleep/awake
- hallucinations
- sleep walking

SELF HARMING BEHAVIOUR

refer to Part 15 – Self harming behaviour

Does the individual

- talk in their sleep
- snore
- grind their teeth
- appear to masturbate
- obviously masturbate

Part 6: Life Experiences

| Has the individual disclosed any of the following to any family member? | yes/no |

| Does the patient believe disclosure will be damaging to any/all family members? | yes/no |

Patient has stated	physical abuse has occurred
Does the family know/believe	physical abuse has occurred
Does the care team have reason to believe	physical abuse has occurred

Patient has stated	emotional abuse has occurred
Does the family know/believe	emotional abuse has occurred
Does the care team have reason to believe	emotional abuse has occurred

Patient has stated	sexual abuse has occurred
Does the family know/believe	sexual abuse has occurred
Does the care team have reason to believe	sexual abuse has occurred

Individual has stated abuser's was/were	• family member(s) • person(s) known to family • person(s) unknown to individual or individual's family • younger/older than victim at the time

Individual was witness to	physical/emotional/sexual abuse
	  ◦ towards whom?
	  ◦ how old? (witness/abuser/abused)
	  ◦ for how long?

Disclosure has taken place to police	yes/no
Abuser went to court	outcome
Abuser deceased	• when • how
Accused abuser deceased	• when • how
Individual states	rape(s) has/have occurred
Family know/believe	rape(s) has/have occurred
Care team have reason to believe	rape(s) has/have occurred
Rape case went to court	outcome

Individual states	sexual harassment has occurred
Family know/believe	sexual harassment has occurred
Care team have reason to believe	sexual harassment has occurred
Case went to court	outcome
Individual complains of 'flashbacks'	uses coping strategies (specify)
Staff believe individual has flashbacks	give reasons for belief
Individual has stated difficulty in communicating with	same sex/opposite sex
Care team have observed difficulty in communicating with	same sex/opposite sex
Individual has stated reluctance to communicate with	same sex/opposite sex
Care team have observed a reluctance to communicate with	same sex/opposite sex
Individual refuses to communicate with	same sex/opposite sex

Does the individual appear to be anxious in the presence of

- men in general
- women in general
- men of a specific age/appearance
- women of a specific age/appearance

Does the individual appear to dislike	<ul><li>men in general</li><li>women in general</li><li>men of a specific age/appearance</li><li>women of a specific age/appearance</li></ul>
Does the individual get obviously distressed when	<ul><li>there is shouting in the same room</li><li>they are shouted at</li><li>they witness a violent incident</li><li>they witness a self harm incident</li></ul>
Does the individual express strong views that the world is an unsafe place for	women/children
Does the individual usually wear clothes that disguise	their shape/their appearance
Has the individual a proven record of prostitution (check Part 13)	
In the event of the individual complaining of 'voices', do they appear to follow an 'abusive' pattern?	e.g.: instructive/derogatory about the individual, etc. Is the individual allowed to discuss the voices?

Individual's previous work
experience

- media
- psychiatry
- general medicine
- emergency services
- other (specify)

Armed forces

where/when

It is believed by the current care
team that the individual is at
risk from others due to

- lack of assertion
- past experiences
- current mental state
- poor self esteem
- disinhibited behaviour
- lack of knowledge

The risk is believed to be

- sexual
- financial
- of pregnancy
- of coercion
- to physical health
- to mental health

Individual's parents divorced	• when
	• who the individual lived with
	• whether siblings stayed together
Individual is divorced	
Individual was witness to a major incident	(specify)
Does the individual want anything to change?	current life style/behaviour, etc.

Part 7:   Security Issues

The individual has been

- secluded
  - by choice/imposed
- in solitary (used Rule 43)
  - by choice/imposed

The individual has attempted to abscond/absconded from

- external escort
- an other hospital
- open facility

The individual has attempted to escape/escaped from

- secure facility
- regional secure unit
- prison
- special hospital

The attempt or event was made

alone/with others

How was the attempt/event

prevented/discovered

How was the individual returned?

The individual can be

- verbally aggressive
- abusive (swears at others)

	• shouts at others (swears/does not)
The individual, without cause	• rings emergency alarm(s) • fire alarm(s)
The individual is believed/known to have	telephoned/written to victim/victim's family
The individual is believed/known to have made obscene phone calls	to person(s) known to them/stranger(s)
The individual has	• made hoax calls to emergency services • made hoax bomb calls (state place called) • called the police believing offence(s) committed by other(s)/self
The individual has a high media profile	• due to nature of offence • was previously known to the public through the local/national media
or has become well known due to	• association with another institution • the individual's own use of the media • escape from another institution

The individual has	been refused telephone/mail/ access/ contact with (specify) restricted telephone/mail/ access/contact with (specify) (give reasons)
The individual is a risk to others due to	<ul><li>impulsive behaviour when general demands not met</li><li>sexual demands</li><li>financial demands</li><li>delusional belief(s)</li><li>psychosis</li></ul>
The individual has family/ friends who are proven or suspected of	<ul><li>using/supplying illegal drugs abusing alcohol</li><li>having a history of violent behaviour</li><li>having a history of abusive behaviour</li><li>may assist the individual to infringe the policies/practices/ protocols of the hospital</li><li>may assist the individual to abscond/escape</li><li>are known to the local media/ national media</li></ul>
Assault/murder (in the event of the victim's death)	(give details) <ul><li>what was the relationship (if any) of the victim to the individual</li></ul>

	• are there others recognised to be at significant risk (specify)
Victim(s) details	• sex
	• age
	• appearance
Has any reason been given for the assault/murder?	(specify)
Did it appear intentional/premeditated?	
Was the individual disinhibited at the time?	drink/drugs/psychosis
Is the risk higher when there are other disinhibiting factors?	• depressive illness/suicidal
	• intention
	• drink/drugs
	• alteration in mental state
Current escorting arrangements	• internal
	• external
	• gender mix of escorting staff
	• numbers of escorting staff
	• with use of C&R techniques
	• with mechanical restraints

Part 8: Previous Placements and Treatments

Has the individual been raised by

- birth parents
- foster parents
- adoptive parents
- other (specify)

Has the individual been in

- residential school/secure child facility/ secure youth facility
- youth/secure youth custody
- hostel
- remand centre
- prison
- community care
- psychiatric unit
- closed ward
- regional secure unit
- special hospital

State when/where/why

Previous treatments

- oral anti-psychotic
- depot anti-psychotic
- lithium/other mood stabiliser(s)
- anti-depressant(s)
- anti-convulsant(s)
- analgesics

Are there any major problems with any medication?

allergy/leucopenia, etc. (specify)

Has the individual attended therapy?

- individual
- psychotherapy/group/family
- anger management/anxiety management/assertion training
- art/drama/music
- other (specify)

Part 9:   Significant Events

Possible significant events prior to self harming or aggressive behaviour

Does it appear to be related to any

- particular day of the week
- particular time of the day
- particular time of the night
- particular time of the month
- particular time of the year

Does it correspond to any particular anniversary?

- index offence
- birthday, self or other
- admission date
- bereavement
- tribunal, etc.
- other (specify)

Does it appear related to visits?

- before
- after
- postponed
- cancelled
- delayed
- terminated

If it appears related to visits	by whom

Does it appear related to

- change
- treatment
- therapy session(s)/with whom/when/ where/before/ during/after

Does it appear related to any social event being

- delayed
- postponed
- cancelled

Does it appear to be related to the changes in	the people around them

Does it appear to be in response to

- another individual
- hallucinations
- delusions
- self opinion
- opinion of others
- external influence(s)

Are there any areas that the individual believes significant?

Are there any areas that the staff feel are significant?

Part 10: Social behaviour

The individual

Initiates conversation with	• other patients
	• other inmates
	• doctors
	• nurses
	• other staff
Will reply when addressed	• yes/no
	• monosyllabic/mute
Spends short periods in	own room/main lounge/small lounge
Spends long periods in	own room/main lounge/small lounge
Only leaves own room when prompted	
Attends dining room	• once a day
	• twice a day
	• for all meals
Leaves the ward/wing to	• attend rehabilitation therapy
	• attend education

- go to shop/hairdressers/
  library
- use the recreational facilities

Accepts delay/change/
security policy/ area practice

Communication and social skills during interview

Excessive/deficit   personal space

Use of language

- descriptive/monosyllabic
  (describe)
- tone/volume
- eye contact while
  speaking/listening

Posture   do they appear relaxed/agitated

Use of gesture

At any time during the   (specify)
interview did you feel
threatened or at risk?

What was being discussed
at the time that you felt
threatened/at risk?

Part 11: Recreational Activities

Does the individual take part in any of the following?

- Religious activities
- Folk club
- Live bands
- Disco evening
- Visiting other residents
- Film club
- Multi-gym
- Keep fit
- Bowls
- Swimming
- Tennis
- Football training
- Cricket
- Drama group
- Chess club
- Band/choir practice
- Karaoke
- Relaxation
- Watches television/listens to radio/music
- Arts and crafts
- Reading
- Card/board games
- Computers/computer games

- Beauty/make-up sessions
- Cooking
- Snooker/pool
- Table tennis
- Other (specify)

Part 12: Threat/Fantasy Issues

Have any of the following been identified as either threat or fantasy?

- Arson
- Beat up
- Blind
- Break windows
- Burn a person (fire/acid/other)
- Cause a vehicle to crash
- Derail a train
- Emasculate
- Escape
- Plant a bomb(s)
- Punch
- Rape
- Ring emergency alarms
- Ring fire alarms
- Scar
- Sexually assault
- Shoot
- Stab
- Strangle
- Take hostage(s)
- Telephone emergency services
- Throw furniture

- Kill (without specific method given)
- Torture
- Reference proposed victim(s)
  - male
  - female
  - adult
  - child
  - baby
  - known
  - stranger
  - ethnic group/type
  - named individual(s)
  - type of individual(s) e.g. doctors
- Self harm
  (use classifications contained within Part 15 – Self harming behaviours)
- To commit suicide
  (use classifications contained within Part 15 – Self harming behaviours)
- To refuse psychiatric prescription
- To refuse medical prescription

Part 13:   Sexual Issues

Is the individual disinhibited
due to current mental state?

Does the individual offer to
participate in sexual activity with

- other residents
- care team members
- people not known to the individual
- same sex
- opposite sex
- either sex

Does the individual ask for
anything in return for sexual
activity?

Has the individual a proven
record of prostitution?

Does the individual masturbate
in a public area?

Does the individual masturbate
in front of individual people?

Does the individual appear to
realise that this is not the social
norm?

Has the individual a history of obsessive behaviour relating to another person(s)?
NB: sometimes referred to as stalking.

Has this been by	telephone/letters/physically following
Age of victim(s)	male(s)/female(s)
Has it been	• someone from a previous relationship • a high media profile personality (specify) • a member of the general public • someone previously known to the individual • someone previously unknown to the individual • someone with whom the individual's current partner was previously involved • someone with whom the individual's ex-partner is currently involved
Has it always been	the same victim(s)/new victim(s)
Have they made themselves known to the victim	by letter/telephone/in person

Have they threatened	• by letter/telephone/in person
	• sexually
	• violence
Have they been	arrested/cautioned/charged/ convicted (specify)

Has the individual given any reason(s) for their behaviour?

Gender

Does the individual express the desire to be of the opposite sex?

Has the individual lived as a member of the opposite sex?

Has the individual attempted to change sex?	• with counselling
	• without counselling
	• with prescribed treatments
	• without prescribed treatments

Does the individual intend to have sexual realignment surgery?

Is sexual realignment surgery	planned/agreed upon

Has the individual started sexual realignment surgery?

Has the individual completed sexual realignment surgery?

Is the individual satisfied with the outcome of sexual realignment surgery?

Is the individual content to live as a member of the opposite sex for the rest of their life?

Part 14: Loss/Bereavement

DEATH OF AN ADULT

- lover male/female
- friend male/female
  - ○ childhood friend(s)
- common law partner male/female
- sibling male/female
- twin sibling male/female
- husband/wife
- mother/father
- foster mother/father
- adoptive mother/father
- grandmother/father maternal
- grandmother/father paternal
- other blood relatives (specify)

How old was the person who died?

How old was the individual when they were bereaved?

Multiple losses within   1 year/2–5 years (specify)

Cause of death	• accident
	• genetic disorder
	• sudden onset/brief illness (specify)
	• long standing illness
	• murder/suicide (specify)
	• sudden death (specify)
The individual found a body	relative/stranger/friend (specify)
The individual found a suicide	relative/stranger/friend (specify)
The individual was witness to	a fatal accident/suicide (specify)
The witness was involved in an accident with fatalities	yes/no
The individual was involved in a suicide pact	yes/no
The individual survived a suicide pact	yes/no
The individual allegedly assisted another in a suicide attempt	yes/no
The individual admits assisting another in a suicide attempt	yes/no
The individual allegedly assisted in a successful suicide	yes/no
The individual admits assisting in a successful suicide	yes/no
Individual identified a body	yes/no
Individual has attended	funeral(s)/cremation(s)

Individual has used support service	CRUSE/Hospice/The London Lighthouse/SANDS/Terrence Higgins Trust/other (specify)
Within the grieving process it is suspected that the individual has not reached acceptance	specify reason(s)

DEATH OF A CHILD

Parentage of child(ren)	<ul><li>unknown/known</li><li>as a result of rape/sex abuse (specify stranger/family member)</li><li>prostitution</li></ul>
Number of pregnancies	
Number of miscarriages	how/when during pregnancy/why
Number of terminations	how/when during pregnancy/why
Infertility	cause/duration
Fertility treatment	how many attempts/where
Stillbirth(s)	when/cause/whether seen
Live birth(s)	number/sex(es)
Diagnosed puerperal psychosis/ depression	treated/when/where

Separating after delivery	less than 12 months/more than 12 months (specify reason)
Sudden Infant Death Syndrome	age of child(ren)/parent
Death of child(ren) under 2	age of child(ren)/parent
Cause of death	• accident (specify)
	• genetic/birth accident (specify)
	• sudden death (specify)
	• long standing/short illness (specify)
	• recognized cause (specify)
	• murder (specify)

Death of a child(ren) under 10	age of child(ren)/parent
under 16	age of child(ren)/parent
under 20	age of child(ren)/parent
over 21	age of child(ren)/parent
Cause of death	• accident (specify)
	• genetic/birth accident (specify)
	• sudden death (specify)
	• long standing/short illness (specify)
	• recognised cause (specify)
	• murder/suicide (specify)

Disabled child(ren)	physically/mentally

Age of parent at birth of child(ren)	
What degree of handicap?	(specify)
Who supplied care?	for how long
Did carer change?	when/why/for how long
Assisted child(ren) to die	alone/with others (specify) age of parent/child(ren)
Individual believed child(ren)	• was/were ill • was terminal
Individual believed to have made child(ren) ill	yes/no
Individual proven to have made child(ren) ill	how/outcome
Individual alleged/proven to have	• emotionally/physically/ sexually abused • been unintentionally/wilfully neglectful of child(ren)
REDUNDANCY	(specify, including length of service and position held) number if more than once
Subsequent life changes	• specify, including financial issues • house repossession • separation from partner/children • relocation from local/family support
Any other significant information	

Part 15: Self Harming Behaviours

W	height as a method of causing self harm	52
X	self stabbing	52
Y	Refusing treatment for medical condition and by their action/action causing medical condition to alter requiring intervention	52
Z	Insertion of foreign body (ies) into ears, nose and throat	53

A Skin damage caused by lacerations

A1	superficial scratches, no treatment required
A2	scratches requiring cleaning, no dressing required
A3	minor lacerations requiring cleaning and a dry dressing
A4	moderate lacerations requiring skin closures and a dry dressing
A5	lacerations requiring skin sutures and a dressing
A6	lacerations requiring layered suturing and dressing
A7	lacerations requiring tendon and/or nerve repair

B Headbanging

B1	headbanging, no obvious injury
B2	headbanging, causing bruising / swelling
B3	headbanging, breaking the skin, requiring cleaning
B4	headbanging, breaking the skin, requiring cleaning and dry dressing
B5	headbanging, breaking the skin, requiring sutures
B6	headbanging, requiring neuro-observations
B7	headbanging until consciousness impaired

C   Hair pulling

C1	pulling out hair, small strands
C2	pulling out hair, large strands
C3	pulling out hair, causing scalp to bleed
C4	pulling out hair, causing scalp to bleed, noticeable bald patches
C5	pulling out hair, more than 50% bald

D   Burns using cigarettes

D1	isolated single cigarette burns
D2	multiple cigarette burns
D3	cigarette burns over small area causing raw area (less than 1 inch)
D4	cigarette burns over large area causing raw area (more than 1 inch)

E   Other burns and scalds

E1	used boiling fluids to cause scalds, minor damage, no treatment required
E2	used boiling fluids to cause scalds, treatment required
E3	used boiling fluids to cause scalds, treatment required in general hospital
E4	used boiling fluids to cause scalds, plastic surgery required
E5	set fire to clothing, burns require treatment
E6	used friction to cause skin damage
E7	used flammable liquids to cause fire, with intent to cause self injury

E8   use of radiators or hot pipe with intent to cause skin damage

F   Damage to eye(s)

F1   hitting own eye(s) causing redness

F2   hitting own eye(s) causing bruising

F3   attempting to insert foreign body(ies) into own eye(s)/eyelid(s)

F4   actually insering foreign body(ies) into own eye(s)/eyelid(s)

F5   attempting to remove eye(s) from socket(s)

F6   actually removing eye(s) from socket(s)

F7   damaging eye(s) further after removing from socket(s)

F8   single cigarette burn to eyelid causing swelling

F9   single cigarette burn to eyelid causing eye to close

F10   single cigarette burn to eyelid requiring ophthalmic referral

F11   multiple cigarette burns to eyelid causing swelling

F12   multiple cigarette burns to eyelid causing eye to close

F13   multiple cigarette burns to eyelid requiring ophthalmic referral

F14   burn to the eye surface requiring ophthalmic referral

F15   introducing toxic liquids into eye(s)

F16   introducing toxic solids/powders into eye(s)

G   Insertion of foreign bodies

G1	inserting foreign body(ies) into the skin
G2	inserting foreign body(ies) into the laceration/wound
G3	inserting foreign body(ies) into the vagina (whether to cause damage to the vagina or not)
G4	inserting foreign body(ies) into the anus (whether to cause damage to the anus or not)
G5	swallowing foreign body(ies), no intervention required
G6	swallowing foreign body(ies), intervention required
G7	swallowing foreign body(ies), surgery required
G8	inserting foreign body(ies) into the urethra (whether to cause injury or not)

H   Use of ligatures

H1	tied ligature around neck, no breathing impairment
H2	tied ligature around neck, breathing impaired
H3	tied ligature around neck, used tool to tighten further
H4	tied ligature around neck, resuscitation required

I   Attempted drowning

I1	attempted to drown themselves within a residential setting
I2	attempted to drown themselves outside of a residential setting
I3	attempted to drown themselves by jumping from a height into water

J Attempted asphyxiation

J1   attempted to asphyxiate themselves using a plastic bag

J2   attempted to asphyxiate themselves using gas

J3   attempted to asphyxiate themselves using carbon monoxide

K Attempted overdosing and ingestion of toxic substances

K1   attempted to overdose using prescription medication

K2   attempted to overdose using non-prescription medication

K3   attempted to overdose using a combination of prescription and non-prescription medication

K4   attempted to overdose using illegal drugs

K4   attempted to overdose using any medication/drugs and alcohol

K6   attempted to ingest toxic substance(s)

K7   actually ingested toxic substance(s)

L Refusing diets/fluid

L1   refusing solid food for less than 1 week

L2   refusing solid food for more than 1 week

L3   refusing dietary supplements

L4   refusing fluids for less than 2 days

L5   refusing fluids for more than 2 days

L6   has required intravenous rehydration

M   Use of traffic or trains in a dangerous manner

M1   Attempted to run out into traffic

M2   actually ran out into traffic

M3   attempted to get in front of a moving train

M4   actually got in front of a moving train

M5   attempted to leave a moving vehicle

M6   actually left a moving vehicle causing self harm

N   Use of firearms

N1   attempted to use a firearm to cause self injury

N2   actually used a firearm to cause self injury

O   Attempted use of electricity to cause self harm

O1   attempted to use electricity to cause self injury

O2   actually used electricity to cause self injury

P   Use of known allergens to cause self harm

P1   attempted to use known allergens to cause self harm

P2   actually used known allergens to cause self harm

Q   Hitting inanimate objects with hands

Q1   hitting inanimate object(s) with hand(s) causing
                       redness

Q2   hitting inanimate object(s) with hand(s) causing
                       swelling and discolouration

Q3   hitting inanimate object(s) with hand(s) requiring
                       X-ray to exclude fracture

Q4   hitting inanimate object(s) with hand(s) requiring treatment for tissue / bone damage

R   Re-opening of previous injury site

R1   re-opened previous injury site, no treatment required

R2   re-opened previous injury site, cleaning and dry dressing required

R3   re-opened previous injury site, adhesive skin closures required

R4   re-opened previous injury site, new skin sutures required

R5   re-opened previous injury site, causing further damage requiring skin suturing

R6   re-opened previous injury site, causing further damage requiring layered suturing

R7   re-opened previous injury site, requiring nerve / tendon repair

S   Injuries to the penis

S1   superficial scratch(es) to penis, no treatment required

S2   laceration(s) to penis, dry dressing required

S3   laceration(s)to penis, skin sutures required

S4   laceration(s) to penis, referral to plastic surgeon / urologist required

S5   constricting/elastic material put around penis

S6   foreign body(ies) inserted into the penis (not the urethra)

S7	swelling/trauma to the penis caused by frequent/constant friction
S8	damage to fraenum, bleeding observed
S9	damage to fraenum, intervention required

T   Injuries to scrotum and testicles

T1	superficial scratch(es) to scrotum, no treatment required
T2	laceration(s) to scrotum, dry dressing required
T3	laceration(s) to scrotum, closure of injury(ies) required
T4	foreign body(ies) inserted into scrotum
T5	lacerated scrotum and exposed testicle(s)
T6	lacerated scrotum, brought testicle(s) outside scrotal sac
T7	removed testicle(s) from the scrotal sac and caused further damage to testicle(s)
T8	removed testicle(s) from scrotal sac and detached from body
T9	hit testicle(s) until red
T10	hit testicle(s), bruising observed
T11	hit testicle(s) until haematoma observed, treatment required

Note: Please check Category G for insertion injury(ies) and Category R for re-opening of previous injuries

U Abrasive materials

U1   used abrasive material to cause redness to skin, no treatment required

U2   used abrasive material to cause superficial grazing, no treatment required

U3   used abrasive material to cause grazing requiring cleaning

U4   used abrasive material to cause grazing requiring cleaning and a dry dressing

U5   used abrasive material to require consultation with plastic surgeon, whether treatment follow or not

V Skin damage caused by biting

V1   bit themselves, causing redness

V2   bit themselves, causing bruising

V3   bit themselves, breaking the skin, no treatment required

V4   bit themselves, cleaning and dry dressing required

V5   bit themselves, consultation with plastic surgeon required

V6   bit themselves, removing a piece of tissue with their teeth

W Height as a method of causing self-harm

W1   jumped out of window

W2   jumped off building

W3   jumped sown stairwell

X   Self stabbing

X1	Stabbed themselves causing superficial puncture wound(s), no treatment required.
X2	Stabbed themselves causing shallow puncture wound(s), dry dressing required
X3	Stabbed themselves causing puncture wound(s), requiring pressure bandage
X4	Stabbed themselves causing puncture wound(s) requiring surgical assessment
X5	Stabbed themselves causing puncture wound(s) requiring surgical treatment
X6	Stabbed themselves causing puncture wound(s) requiring repair under anaesthetic

Y   Refusing treatment for medical treatment

Y1	Refused treatment for a diagnosed medical condition, no action required
Y2	Refused treatment for a diagnosed medical condition, alternative treatment required
Y3	Refused treatment for a diagnosed medical condition, urgent treatment required
Y4	Refused treatment for a diagnosed medical condition, emergency treatment in general hospital required
Y5	By the action/inaction of the individual their diagnosed medical condition altered and further treatment was required
Y6	By the action/inaction of the individual their diagnosed medical condition altered and they required urgent treatment

Y7   By the action/inaction of the individual their diagnosed medical condition worsened to such a degree they needed emergency treatment in a general hospital

Z Insertion of foreign body(ies) into ears, nose and throat

Z1   Inserted foreign body(ies) into ear(s), requiring medical intervention

Z2   Inserted foreign body(ies) into ear(s) requiring ENT referral

Z3   Inserted foreign body(ies) into nose, requiring medical intervention

Z4   Inserted foreign body(ies) nose, requiring ENT referral

Z5   Inserted foreign body(ies) into throat requiring medical inervention

Z6   Inserted foreign body(ies) into nose, requiring emergency treatment/resuscitation

Z7   Inserted foreign body(ies) into nose and throat, requiring emergency treatment/ resuscitation

Part 16: Hostage Taking History

Did the individual prevent a person/people leaving the area?

Did the individual take/hold hostage(s)?

Did the individual attempted to take hostage(s) into a new area?

Did the individual act alone in taking hostage(s)?

Did the individual display a weapon or weapons?	state type(s) of weapon(s)
Did the individual use a weapon or weapons?	state type(s) of weapon(s)
Did the individual immobilise the hostage(s)?	state method(s) of immobilisation employed
Did the individual injure the hostage(s)?	
Did any/all of the hostages die?	how and at what point during the incident

What were the individual's demands/grievances?

Was the situation prevented from escalating?	(give details)

How was the situation finally resolved?

Did the individual attempt suicide at any time during the hostage incident?

Did the individual attempt suicide within 24 hours of the incident's resolution?

Did the hostage taking incident occur during the committing of another crime?

Where did the hostage incident take place? was it in a secure environment, e.g. prison (specify)

Were the hostages

- male
- female
- adult (age)
- child (age)
- baby (age)
- a combination of any of the above (specify)

Part 17: Eating Issues

Does the individual

- binge/vomit

- misuse laxatives/diuretics/enemas

Does the individual limit the type of dietary intake, e.g. crackers and squash only?

Does the individual perceive their whole body to be fat or just parts, e.g. hips and thighs?

Does the individual weigh/measure themselves more than once a week?

Does the individual eat in public?

Is there evidence of

hypotension/hypothermia/ bradycardia/anaemia/ constipation/dry skin/new soft body hair?

Does the individual complain of a physical cause for not eating?

Has this been investigated, to what outcome?

Does the individual express a
fear of becoming fat?

Does the individual have regular
episodes of binge eating?

Does the individual prevent
weight gain by

self induced vomiting/misuse of
laxatives/diuretics/enemas/other
medication/fasting

Does the individual binge on a
particular type of food?

Does the individual use a
marker, e.g. tomato juice?

Can the individual vomit at will?

Is the individual always
prepared for binging?

Does the individual take
excessive exercise?

Does the individual exercise
alone?

Does the individual dilute fluids
excessively, e.g. use a
teaspoonful of soup powder
instead of a whole sachet?

Does the individual spit out
food instead of swallowing?

Does the individual always
vomit after eating?

Does the individual cook for
others but not eat with them?

Will the individual drink dietary
supplements?

Does the individual believe food
is contaminated/poisoned?

Does the individual follow a
specific diet, e.g. vegan/kosher?

Has the individual used appetite
suppressors, e.g. Tenuate
Dospan?

Has the individual used meal
substitutes, e.g. low calorie
drinks/meals?

Part 18: Arson

The individual

Set fire alone

Set fire with others

Called fire brigade

Did not call fire brigade

Called other emergency services

Left the scene immediately   when the fire brigade arrived/after the fire was extinguished

Returned to the fire scene   later/and set another fire

Attitude towards their own personal risk during fire setting

Attitude towards the risk to others

Attitude towards the damage caused

Whether the fire is finished (do they intend to return to the scene for the purpose of further fire setting?)

Does the individual know why they set the fire?

Are they willing/able to discuss the reason for setting the fire(s)?

What emotion did the individual feel	before/during/after the act

Was the emotion before the act	sudden/sustained

Does the individual express feelings of	fear/guilt/anger/revenge/depression/anxiety/other (specify)

Did the individual feel	sexually excited/gratified at any time
Did the individual	orgasm/ejaculate at any time

Did the individual feel in control at any time?

Did the individual feel out of control at any time?

Did the individual attempt to extinguish the fire	by urinating on it/or other means (specify)

Was any threat of arson actively attempted?

Was the threat to
- themselves/people known to them/strangers
- property belonging to self/person(s) known/strangers

Was the target of the arson
- house/hostel/communal accommodation/ hospital/ prison/farm/garage/shed/ other building(s) (specify)
- bedroom/lounge/other room (specify)
- occupied/unoccupied at the time of the fire setting

Was the individual aware of the state of occupation at the time of the fire setting?

Was the fire setting

during the day/night

Was the fire started with

matches/lighter/cigarette/ flammable liquid/flammable solids, e.g. fire lighters, candle/other (specify)

Was the initial target

rubbish in a bin/bedding/ curtains/ furniture/paper/ materials in a car/other (specify)

Was an incendiary device attached to a timer used to start the fire?

Did the individual send an incendiary device through the post?

Did the individual conceal an incendiary device in a public place, e.g.: department store

Number of fires known to have been set/claimed to have been set/admitted to have been set

Is there any suggestion that the individual has set a fire in their current/previous placement that was not proven to have been set by them?

Has the individual restricted their fire setting to targets where little major damage is likely?

Has the nature of the targets chosen changed to include those where risk to property/persons has become a possibility?

Has there been an escalation in the severity of the fire setting?

Has there been an escalation in the frequency of the acts of fire setting?

Has the individual been injured
during the fire setting?

Has the individual stated that
they intended to end their life in
the fire?

Notes

Notes

Notes